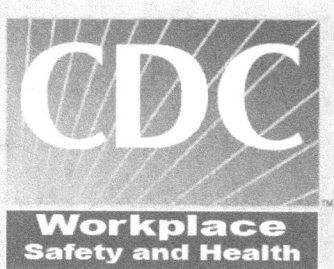

Workplace Safety and Health

Evaluation of Health Effects of a Chlorine Gas Release in a Poultry Processing Plant — Arkansas

Francisco Meza, MD, MPH
Charles Mueller, MS
Bradley King, MPH, CIH

Health Hazard Evaluation Report
HETA 2011-0128-3166
September 2012
Revised February 2013

DEPARTMENT OF HEALTH AND HUMAN SERVICES
Centers for Disease Control and Prevention

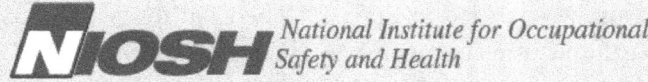 National Institute for Occupational Safety and Health

The employer shall post a copy of this report for a period of 30 calendar days at or near the workplace(s) of affected employees. The employer shall take steps to insure that the posted determinations are not altered, defaced, or covered by other material during such period. [37 FR 23640, November 7, 1972, as amended at 45 FR 2653, January 14, 1980].

Revision Summary: The authors incorrectly identified that a Spanish-speaking employee poured sodium hypochlorite into a 55-gallon drum containing residual acidic antimicrobial solution, causing a chlorine gas release. The Spanish-speaking employee retrieved a 55-gallon drum containing residual acidic antrimicrobial solution. The drum was labeled in English. The English-speaking supervisor mixed the sodium hypochlorite into the 55-gallon drum containing residual acidic antimicrobial solution, but did not read the label.

CONTENTS

ABBREVIATIONS

ACGIH®	American Conference of Governmental Industrial Hygienists
CFR	Code of Federal Regulations
ECRHS	European Community Respiratory Health Survey
FEV1	Forced expiratory volume in 1 second
mg/m³	Milligrams per cubic meter of air
mL	Milliliter
NAICS	North American Industry Classification System
NIOSH	National Institute for Occupational Safety and Health
OEL	Occupational exposure limit
OSHA	Occupational Safety and Health Administration
ppm	Parts per million
PEL	Permissible exposure limit
PTSD	Posttraumatic stress disorder
RADS	Reactive airway dysfunction syndrome
REL	Recommended exposure limit
STEL	Short-term exposure limit
TLV®	Threshold limit value
TWA	Time-weighted average
WEEL™	Workplace environmental exposure level

Highlights of the NIOSH Health Hazard Evaluation

The National Institute for Occupational Safety and Health (NIOSH) received a request for a health hazard evaluation at a poultry processing plant in Arkansas. The Occupational Safety and Health Administration submitted the request to determine health outcomes of an unintentional chlorine gas release in June 2011. NIOSH investigators visited the plant in June 2011, November 2011, and January 2012.

What NIOSH Did

- We investigated the causes of the chlorine gas release.

- We interviewed 545 employees during part or all of our evaluation.

- We interviewed employees about exposure to the chlorine gas. Interviews were done in English, Spanish, and Marshallese.

- We asked about acute symptoms in the days following the chlorine gas release.

- We interviewed employees 4 months after the chlorine gas release. We wanted to see if they had symptoms of asthma or posttraumatic stress disorder.

- Employees who reported symptoms of asthma 4 months after the chlorine gas release had a breathing test done six months after the release. This test was used to see if they had reactive airway dysfunction syndrome. This condition is asthma caused by a single, high exposure to an irritant such as chlorine.

What NIOSH Found

- Several factors led to the chlorine gas release. Among them were labeling in English only, lack of literacy in English, storage of incompatible chemicals in similar containers, and failure to read labels.

- One hundred sixteen (21%) participants had asthma symptoms 4 months after the release. Of these, three participants had breathing tests consistent with reactive airway dysfunction syndrome 6 months after the release.

- One hundred six (19%) participants had posttraumatic stress disorder symptoms 4 months after the release.

What Managers Can Do

- Find unique fittings that will prevent connections from the filling station to containers that should not be filled with sodium hypochlorite.

- Keep incompatible chemicals in different sized or different colored barrels to help keep from them being mixed up.

- Properly label containers in English, Spanish, and Marshallese. Labels should be written to meet at a reading level that all employees can understand.

HIGHLIGHTS OF THE NIOSH HEALTH HAZARD EVALUATION (CONTINUED)

- Teach employees about chemical hazards. This should be done in the employees' native language.

- Train employees on the proper exit routes from the plant.

- Refer employees who are still experiencing symptoms to a trained healthcare provider. Employees who still have respiratory symptoms should be seen by a pulmonologist. Employees who have psychological symptoms should see a psychologist. Employees with other work-related symptoms should seek care from an occupational health physician.

What Employees Can Do

- Tell managers about any safety and health concerns that you may have about your workplace.

- Read labels on all chemicals.

- Participate in all safety training that your employer offers.

- Tell your supervisor or the plant health clinic if you are still having any physical or psychological symptoms related to the chlorine gas release. They can help you get the proper care.

SUMMARY

A large release of chlorine gas resulted from the unintentional mixing of sodium hypochlorite solution and an acidic antimicrobial used at this poultry processing plant. Several factors led to the chlorine gas release. Among them were labeling in English only, lack of literacy in English, storage of incompatible chemicals in similar containers, and failure to read labels. Three employees developed RADS, and more than 100 had symptoms of PTSD.

NIOSH received a request for technical assistance from OSHA to evaluate employee health effects after a chlorine gas release in a poultry processing plant in Arkansas. On the morning of June 27, 2011, human error resulted in the mixing of an acidic solution of Fresh FX, an antimicrobial used in poultry processing, with a sodium hypochlorite solution. This mixing of chemicals caused a release of chlorine gas into the plant. About 600 employees who were at work at the time of the release were evacuated.

We made three site visits to evaluate the employees who were at work on the morning of the release. Five hundred forty-five employees participated in part or all of our evaluation. Of those who participated in our evaluation, 195 reported seeking medical care, 152 reported being hospitalized, and the company reported that 5 were admitted to intensive care units immediately after the incident.

On our first site visit in June 2011, we spoke with an employee involved in the chlorine release and the managers about what led to the event. We administered questionnaires about medical history and symptoms in the days following the incident to employees in Spanish, English, and Marshallese. On the second site visit in November 2011, we evaluated participants for symptoms of asthma (because a single high level exposure to an irritant like chlorine can cause a type of asthma called RADS) and PTSD approximately 4 months after the release. On our third site visit in January 2012, we did spirometry and methacholine challenge tests on participants who reported asthma symptoms at the second site visit, but had no history of asthma prior to the release.

Five hundred twenty-three participants were present at the first site visit and at work on the morning of the chlorine release. An additional 22 were later identified as present the morning of the chlorine release but not during the first site visit. Of the 545 participants, 60% were female, 17% primarily spoke English, 68% primarily spoke Spanish, 12% primarily spoke Marshallese, and 3% spoke other languages. Eleven percent of participants were current smokers, and 6% reported a history of asthma. Strength of chlorine odor was used as a surrogate for intensity of exposure. Of the 542 participants who responded to the question of whether or not they smelled chlorine, 29% reported not smelling chlorine, and 22% reported a light odor, 7% a moderate odor, and 42% a strong odor.

Of the 523 participants who were present at the first visit, 213 (41%) reported a strong chlorine odor. Their most commonly reported symptoms within 24 hours of the chlorine release were burning throat, headache, burning eyes, and cough. Headache, burning throat, and cough were the most common symptoms reported 3–5 days post-release by those reporting a strong chlorine odor.

Two hundred forty-five participants (47%) present at the first site visit reported lower respiratory tract symptoms (cough, shortness of breath, chest tightness, or wheeze). These 245 plus 22 additional participants who had not yet returned to work at the time of our first site visit were asked to complete the asthma symptoms questionnaire during the second site visit. Of the 240 who did so, 116 (48%) had one or more asthma symptoms in the 2 weeks prior to that site visit.

Overall, 106 (22%) of 493 participants at the second site visit reported symptoms consistent with PTSD approximately 4 months after the release. The prevalence of PTSD symptoms increased with increasing strength of reported chlorine odor (from 4% among those who reported not smelling chlorine to 37% among those reporting a strong odor of chlorine, P<0.01).

At the third site visit we did spirometry on 101 subjects who reported asthma symptoms at the second site visit and had no history of asthma prior to the release. Methacholine challenge testing was done on 78 participants with a forced expiratory volume at 1 second at or above 70% (this means they did not have significant obstruction) and no medical contraindications for testing. Three had borderline bronchial hyperreactivity, two had mild bronchial hyperreactivity, and one had moderate to severe bronchial hyperreactivity. Mild, moderate, and severe bronchial hyperreactivity are consistent with RADS, or asthma.

The unintentional release of chlorine gas at this plant posed a serious health hazard to employees. Three employees developed RADS, and more than 100 developed symptoms of PTSD.

Keywords: NAICS 311615 (Poultry Processing), asthma, reactive airways dysfunction syndrome, posttraumatic stress disorder, chlorine

INTRODUCTION

NIOSH received a request from OSHA to evaluate employee health effects after a chlorine gas release in a poultry processing plant in Arkansas. The plant prepared poultry for consumption from slaughtering through processing, seasoning, and packaging. A sodium hypochlorite solution was often used for disinfection. On the morning of June 27, 2011, an employee inadvertently mixed an acidic solution of Fresh FX, an antimicrobial, with a hypochlorite solution, releasing chlorine gas into the plant. About 600 employees were at work and were evacuated. Of those who participated in our evaluation, 195 reported seeking medical care, 152 reported being hospitalized, and the company reported that 5 were admitted to intensive care units immediately after the incident.

Background

Chlorine, Reactive Airway Dysfunction Syndrome, and Posttraumatic Stress Disorder

Chlorine is a greenish-yellow gas. It has a strong, pungent smell, with an odor threshold of approximately 0.3–0.5 ppm. Chlorine is moderately water soluble, so it can enter the upper and lower respiratory tract, and often affects mucous membranes, eyes, and the lower respiratory tract. It forms hydrochloric and hypochlorous acid, two highly irritating compounds, upon contact with water in the eyes, mucous membranes, and lower respiratory tract [Das and Blanc 1993]. A possible long-term effect of a single, high-level chlorine gas exposure is RADS, which is a type of asthma [Shakeri et al. 2008]. Diagnostic criteria for RADS are listed in Appendix A.

Large, unintentional chemical releases can cause anxiety, which may manifest as a range of effects, spanning from an acute stress disorder in the short term to PTSD in the long term. For example, PTSD was documented after a chlorine release from a train derailment in South Carolina [Duncan et al. 2011]. PTSD occurs after a traumatic event that involves actual or threatened death or serious injury or a threat to the physical integrity of self or others [American Psychiatric Association 2000]. The response to the traumatic experience may involve lasting fear and perseveration about the dangers of the event. Diagnostic criteria for PTSD are listed in Appendix A.

First Site Visit (June 29–July 1, 2011)

We met with management and employee representatives, the OSHA compliance officer investigating the incident, and representatives of the local health department to discuss the health hazard evaluation request. We also discussed safety procedures, medical support, and details of the chlorine gas release. We conducted a brief tour of the poultry plant, accompanied by the OSHA compliance officer, paying special attention to how and where the chlorine gas was released. We interviewed one employee directly involved in the release; the other employee involved in the release was not available for interview. We administered questionnaires about past medical history and acute symptoms related to the chlorine release to employees present during our visit. Questionnaires were given in the employees' native language, including Spanish, English, and Marshallese.

Second Site Visit (November 2–4, 2011)

We surveyed two groups of participants, those present and participating during the first visit and an additional group of employees present during the incident but unavailable during the first visit. Questionnaires covered PTSD and asthma symptoms.

We evaluated all participants for symptoms of PTSD. We used the Trauma Screening Questionnaire, a validated questionnaire to screen for symptoms of PTSD [Brewin et al. 2002]. When used in rail crash survivors and crime victims, it had a sensitivity (i.e., correctly identified persons with PTSD) of 76%–86% and specificity (i.e., correctly identified persons without PTSD) of 93%–97% compared to a structured clinical interview [Brewin 2005].

From the first questionnaire, we identified participants who were present at the plant during the chlorine release who reported cough, shortness of breath, chest tightness, or wheeze at 3–5 days after the chlorine release. These participants, plus the employees not available during our first visit, were surveyed to determine if they had symptoms of RADS using modified questions from the ECRHS [Grassi et al. 2003]. Answering yes to any one of these questions is 75% sensitive and 80% specific for being assessed "asthma-like symptomatic," compared with clinical examination, spirometry, and allergy testing.

In addition to the survey items described above, the employees absent during our first site visit but present during the chlorine release were also asked additional items. These included asthma history, strength of chlorine odor, and smoking status.

Third Site Visit (January 9–12, 2012)

We did spirometry on participants who reported asthma symptoms at our second site visit and had no history of asthma prior to the release. The spirometry test measures how well the lungs move air in and out. Because asthma demonstrates intermittent obstruction, spirometry can be normal between attacks. Therefore, we conducted methacholine challenge testing on participants whose forced expiratory volume in 1 second was 70% or greater, which means they did not have significant obstruction. Methacholine causes obstruction in people with bronchial hyperreactivity, indicating they may have asthma. We also administered the modified ECRHS for asthma symptoms that we used at our second site visit, but asked about asthma symptoms in the 2 weeks prior to the testing. An interpreter assisted when needed, and informed consent was obtained. The flow diagram below outlines activities from all three site visits. A detailed description of methacholine challenge testing is in Appendix B.

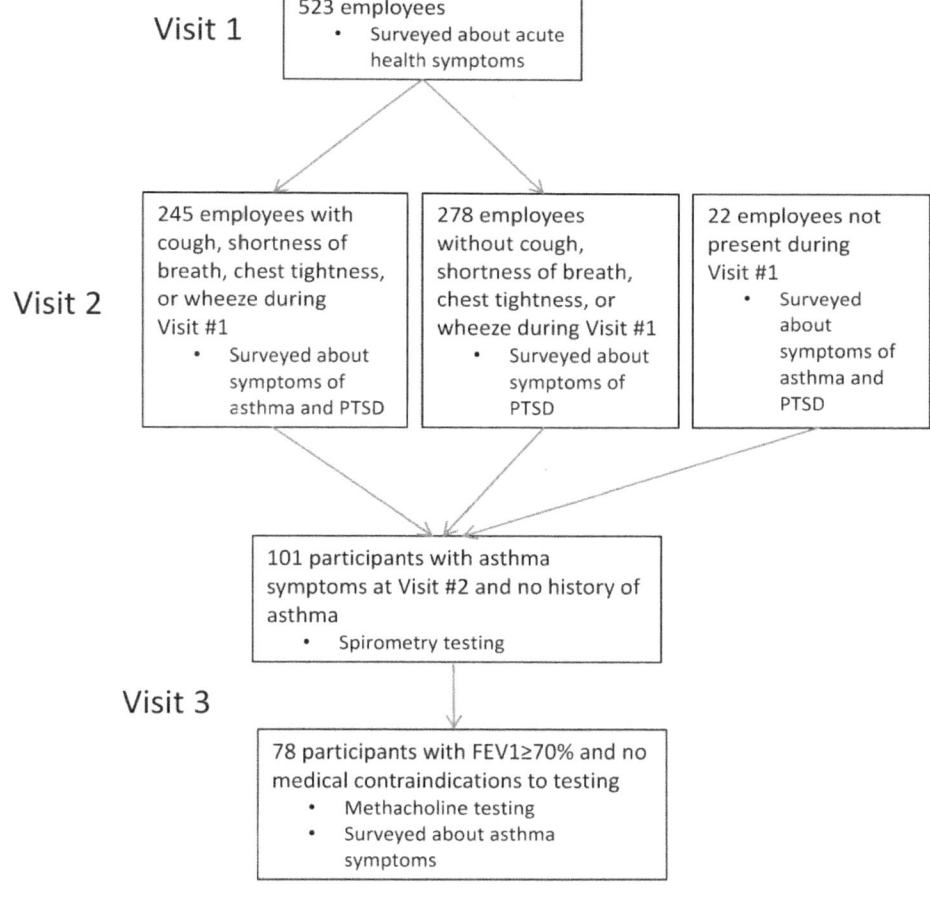

Figure 1. Flow diagram of activities from all three site visits.

Statistical Analysis

All data were analyzed using SAS 9.2 (SAS Institute Inc , Cary, North Carolina). We reported descriptive statistics for demographic characteristics and symptoms of participants. We also did Cochran-Armitage tests for trends to assess the presence of an association between exposure (based on chlorine odor strength) and asthma symptoms and exposure and PTSD symptoms. A P value equal to or less than 0.05 was considered statistically significant.

RESULTS

First Site Visit

Interview

We spoke, in Spanish, with an employee who was directly involved in the chlorine release. He reported that the employee who normally filled the barrel was busy and instructed him to get the barrel so it could be refilled with sodium hypochlorite. He found a nearly empty barrel that was labeled in English only. He was not aware that the barrel contained Fresh FX. The other employee actually dispensed the sodium hypochlorite into the barrel. This employee reported he did not read the label on the drum. Chlorine gas was released immediately. That employee was forced to leave the room immediately and could not shut off the valve, but immediately reported what had happened and the hypochlorite valve was shut off remotely. By then the gas had spread throughout the plant.

Questionnaire

Five hundred twenty-three employees participated in the survey at the first site visit. An additional 22 employees were at work the morning of the chlorine release, but not during the first site visit. Demographic and other characteristics of all 545 participants are shown in Table 1. Sixty percent of survey participants were female, 17% spoke primarily English, 68% spoke primarily Spanish, 12% spoke primarily Marshallese, and 3% spoke other languages. Eleven percent of participants were current smokers, and 6% reported a history of asthma.

Table 1. Characteristics of participants (n=543–545)*

Age (years)	Mean 42 (range:18–72)
	No. (%)
Sex	
Male	219 (40)
Female	326 (60)
Primary Language	
English	91 (17)
Spanish	371 (68)
Marshallese	68 (12)
Other	15 (3)
Smoking Status	
Never	411 (76)
Former	73 (13)
Current	59 (11)
History of asthma	34 (6)

*The number of responses varies because of missing data.

Strength of chlorine odor was used as a surrogate for intensity of exposure (Figure 2). Of the 213 participants who reported a strong odor at the first site visit, burning throat, headache, burning eyes, and cough were the most commonly reported symptoms within 24 hours of the chlorine release (Table 2). For all symptoms, prevalence increased with increasing odor strength.

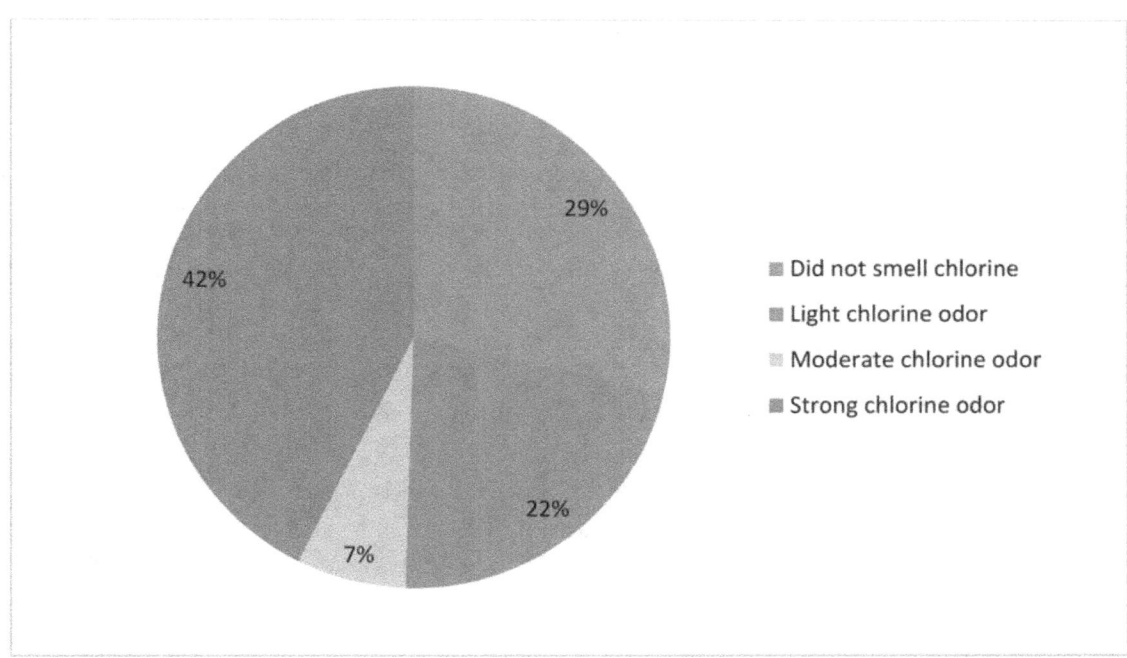

Figure 2. Reported strength of chlorine odor (n=542).

Table 2. Prevalence of reported symptoms among participants within 24 hours of chlorine gas release by self-reported strength of chlorine odor (n=520)*

Symptoms	Strength of Chlorine Odor			
	% None n=154	% Light n=117	% Moderate n=36	% Strong n=213
Mucous membrane				
Burning throat	11	33	56	82
Burning eyes	10	31	50	74
Burning nose	5	21	33	58
Constitutional				
Headache	15	43	61	81
Dizziness/ lightheadedness	6	23	44	63
Chest				
Coughing	8	32	58	72
Shortness of breath	4	12	39	67
Chest pain	5	20	33	66
Chest tightness	6	9	36	56
Chest congestion or phlegm	6	9	31	49
Wheezing in chest	2	6	11	40
Coughing up blood	0	1	0	10
Gastrointestinal				
Nausea	5	13	36	52
Vomiting	2	6	14	25
Skin				
Irritation/pain/burning of skin	3	5	8	26

*Only participants who were present at our first site visit were included.

Headache, burning throat, and cough were the most common symptoms reported 3–5 days post-release (Table 3). For all symptoms, prevalence increased with increasing odor strength. Of those who reported a strong chlorine odor, 69% reported seeking medical care, 58% reported they were hospitalized, and 51% were prescribed medication immediately after the release. In those who experienced no odor, only 4% reported seeking medical care, 3% reported receiving hospital care, and 3% reported being prescribed medication (Figure 3). In addition, many employee questions and comments raised during our evaluation indicated the need for timely and clear risk communication to the employees and staff about what occurred on June 27, 2011.

Table 3. Prevalence of reported symptoms among participants 3 to 5 days after chlorine gas release by self-reported strength of chlorine odor (n=520)*

Symptoms	Strength of Chlorine Odor			
	% None n=154	% Light n=117	% Moderate n=36	% Strong n=213
Mucus membrane				
Burning throat	9	29	39	66
Burning eyes	5	21	31	48
Burning nose	4	17	19	33
Constitutional				
Headache	15	32	42	69
Dizziness/ lightheadedness	5	14	22	47
Chest				
Coughing	8	23	44	64
Shortness of breath	5	16	25	55
Chest pain	5	19	19	53
Chest tightness	5	10	31	46
Chest congestion or phlegm	8	14	25	43
Wheezing in chest	3	4	11	28
Coughing up blood	1	0	0	8
Gastrointestinal				
Nausea	3	9	17	34
Skin				
Irritation/pain/burning of skin	4	7	6	20

*Only participants who were present at our first site visit were included.

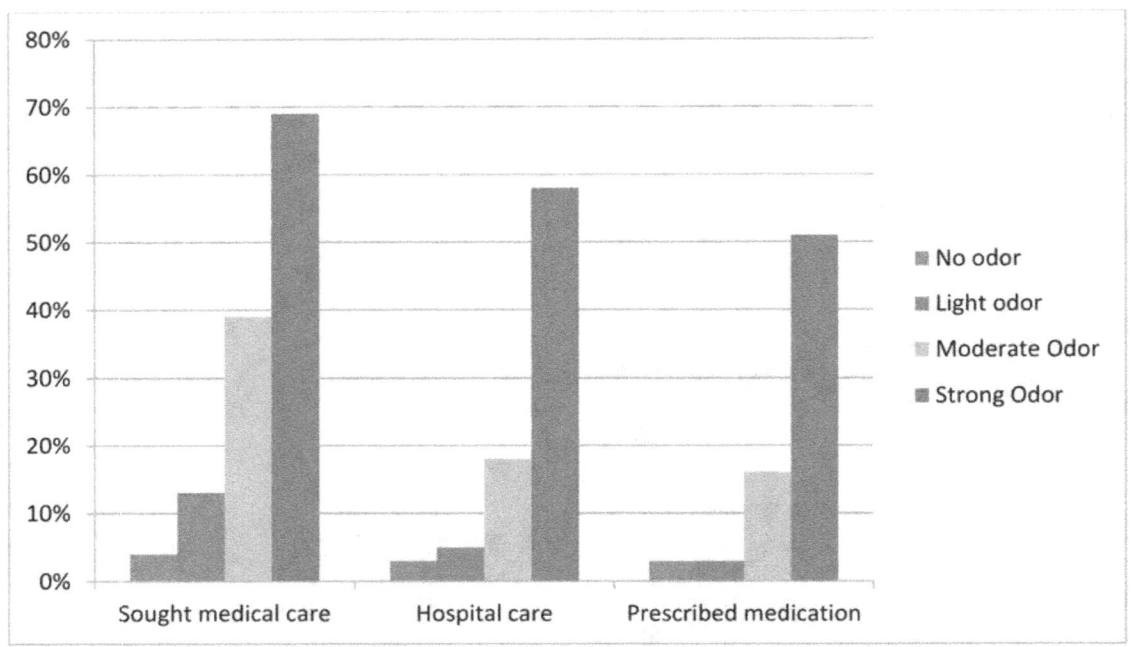

Figure 3. Level of medical care among participants by strength of reported chlorine odor (n=533–541). [The number of responses varies because of missing data.]

Second Site Visit

Post-traumatic Stress Disorder

Twenty-two percent (106/493) of participants reported symptoms consistent with PTSD. The prevalence of PTSD symptoms increased with increasing strength of reported chlorine odor (P<0.01) (Figure 4).

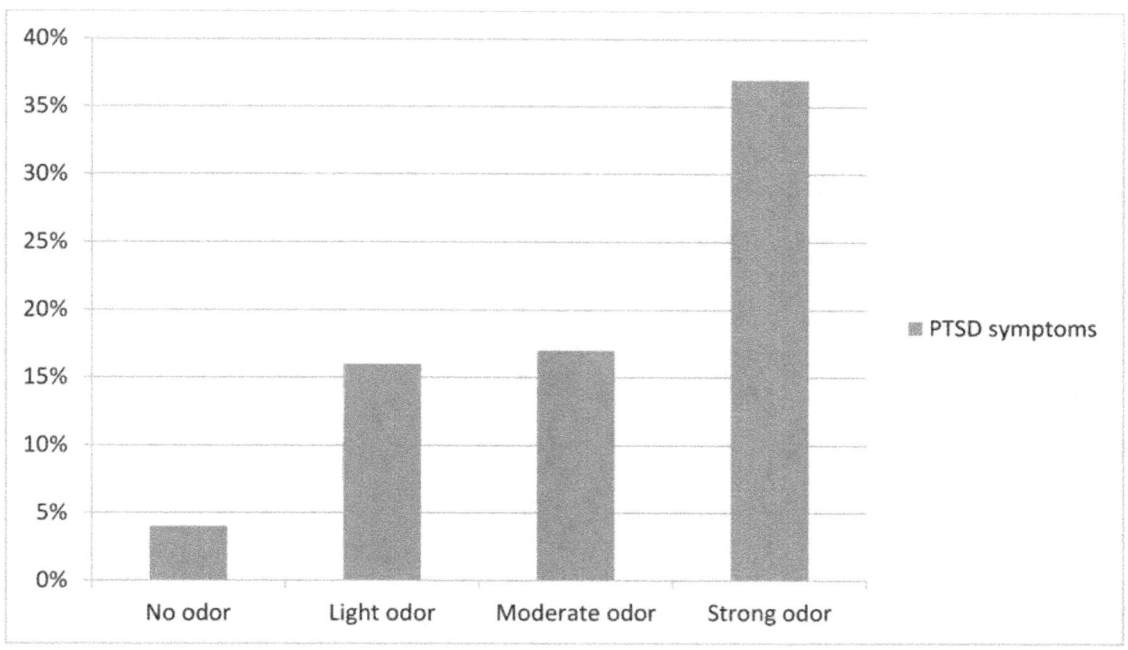

Figure 4. Prevalence of PTSD symptoms by reported chlorine odor strength (n=490).

Reactive Airway Dysfunction Syndrome

Forty-seven percent (245/523) of participants from the first site visit reported one or more respiratory tract symptoms (cough, shortness of breath, chest tightness, wheeze) at 3–5 days post-release. An additional 22 participants who were at work on the day of release but were not present during our first site visit were surveyed in the second site visit. Ninety percent (240/267) of these participants completed the asthma symptoms questionnaire, and of these, 116 (48%) reported one or more asthma symptoms in the 2 weeks prior to the second site visit. The prevalence of asthma symptoms increased with increasing strength of chlorine odor ($P=0.048$) (Figure 5).

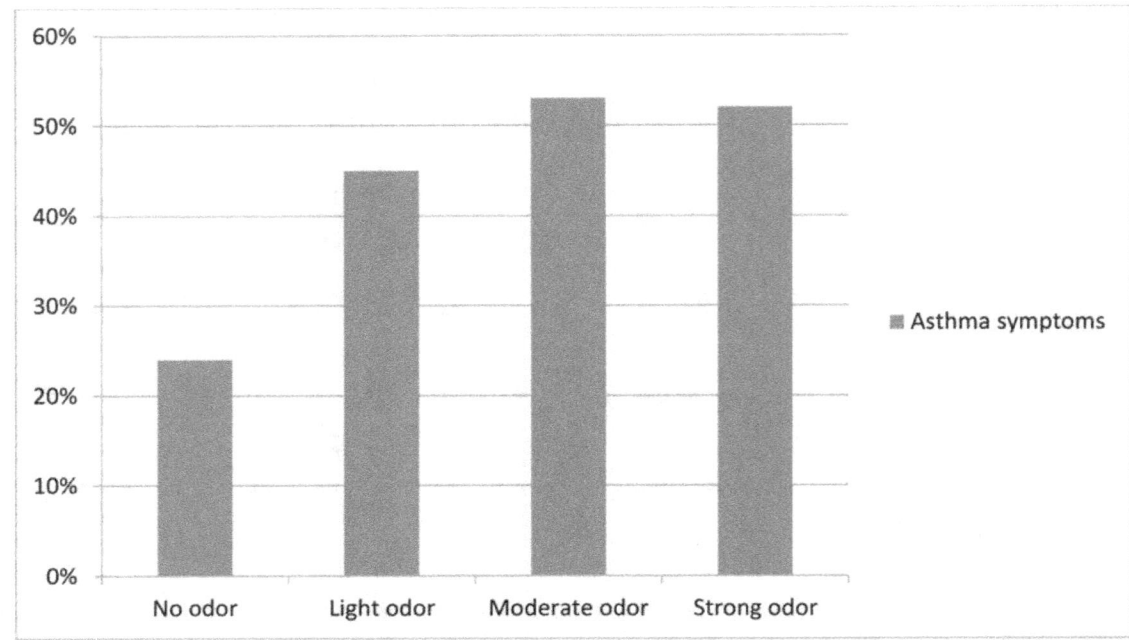

Figure 5. Prevalence of asthma symptoms by reported chlorine odor strength (n=238).

Third Site Visit

Of the 116 participants with asthma symptoms at the second site visit (4 months after the chlorine release), 11 participants had a history of asthma prior to the chlorine release and were excluded from spirometry. One hundred one subjects participated in spirometry. Ninety-four (93%) had normal spirometry, four had a restrictive pattern (RADS normally shows an obstructive pattern), one had low forced expiratory volume in 1 second, and two had uninterpretable results.

Methacholine challenge testing was done on the 78 participants who had no medical contraindications for testing and whose forced expiratory volume in 1 second was 70% or greater. Seventy-two (92%) had a normal test. Three participants had borderline bronchial hyperreactivity, two had mild bronchial hyperreactivity, and one had moderate to severe bronchial hyperreactivity. Mild, moderate, or severe bronchial hyperreactivity is consistent with the diagnosis of RADS.

DISCUSSION

Of 545 employees, 3 developed RADS from this release of chlorine gas, a preventable event. While almost 200 participants sought medical care for their symptoms immediately after the release, and more than 150 reported being hospitalized, including 5 who received intensive care, the vast majority had no evidence of long-lasting respiratory complications. The employees with RADS and borderline RADS need continued medical follow-up by a physician. In one previous study of persons diagnosed with RADS, more than half continued to report symptoms and one third required medication years after their diagnosis [Malo et al. 2009]. RADS has been associated with decreased quality of life and increased depression and anxiety [Malo et al. 2009].

Many employee questions and comments raised during our evaluation indicated the need for timely and clear risk communication to the employees and staff about what occurred on June 27, 2011. In our experience, lack of clear information or a management response that is perceived as unsatisfactory can lead to distortions of information, development of rumors, and unneeded stress and worry among employees. This could contribute to PTSD symptoms. PTSD symptoms affected more than 20% of participants. Because these findings were based on a screening test, and diagnosis of PTSD is done with a psychological or psychiatric clinical evaluation, we believe employees with continuing symptoms should receive medical follow-up to determine if they have clinical PTSD and, if so, get treatment. Bisson found that symptoms can continue for up to 6 years in one-third of people diagnosed with PTSD, decreasing the quality of life for affected individuals [Bisson 2007]. In another chlorine gas release following a train derailment in Graniteville, South Carolina, approximately 48% of respondents reported symptoms of PTSD [Duncan et al. 2011]. The occurrence of fatalities at Graniteville may explain the higher rate of PTSD symptoms than in our evaluation.

Several factors may have contributed to the improper mixing of chemicals that caused the chlorine release in this plant. Among them were the fact that containers were labeled only in English, yet English was not the primary language of most employees, the similarity of containers containing different chemicals, and the failure to read the label. This incident demonstrates the importance of using appropriate languages when communicating in the workplace. This can be challenging given the number and diversity on non-English speaking employees present in the workforce. The Bureau of Labor Statistics reported that the U.S. workforce in animal slaughtering and processing was 38.1% Hispanic or Latino and 8.6% Asian in 2011 [Bureau of Labor Statistics 2011]. The potential for injury due to inadequate attention to foreign language health and safety training extends beyond this industry, with approximately 39 9 million foreign-born residents in the United States; 47.1% are Latino and 51.6% report inability to speak English very well [American Community Survey 2010]. We did not extensively evaluate the training programs at this plant but this information is relevant to all workplaces with employees who are not fluent and/or literate in English.

In addition to language differences, low-level literacy is an impediment to understanding. While we did not formally assess literacy in native language or in English if it was the secondary language, literacy was reported to be low among employees in this plant. The National Assessment of Adult Literacy found that 11 million adults are not literate in English, with 7 million who could not answer simple questions and 4 million who could not take the test because of language barriers [Institute of Education Sciences 2003]. An additional 30 million adults had below basic literacy skills, e.g., skills needed for understanding a television guide or comparing ticket prices. Thus, people with no more than basic literacy skills represent a substantial part of the workforce and often are working in dangerous jobs [U.S. Government Accountability Office 2005; Johnson and Ostendorf 2010]. This situation presents a challenge for employers and for occupational safety and health professionals. Most material safety data sheets used in industry are written at a college reading level, making it difficult to communicate with average employees who are often at a 9th to 12th grade reading level; the problem is compounded when employees do not speak English well or at all [Arcury et al. 2010].

Workplace safety and health training and labeling should be conducted in the specific languages of the workforce. Overcoming the issues of limited English literacy in workers goes beyond providing written training in the appropriate language; it also requires active engagement of employees in hands-on training [Wallerstein 1992]. To decrease communication gaps, training should be interactive, and employees and employers should work together on a health and safety team to analyze and improve workplace policies and programs. You could use your joint labor management safety committee to do this. From a regulatory perspective, OSHA has made changes to the hazard

DISCUSSION (CONTINUED)

communication standard that will be phased in over the next 4 years in accordance with recommendations from the United Nations [OSHA 2012]. These changes establish a standardized international labeling system (the Global Harmonized System of Classification and Labeling of Chemicals) to be used by manufacturers of chemicals. Using symbols and simplified text, its intent is to improve understanding of chemical hazards for all employers and employees regardless of primary language or literacy level.

The findings of this evaluation may have certain limitations. No questionnaires were validated in all three languages, so differences may have occurred as a result of translations. One hundred one subjects had spirometry, but only 78 subjects had methacholine challenge testing. Therefore, the incidence of RADS may be underestimated.

CONCLUSIONS

The unintentional release of chlorine gas at this plant posed a serious health hazard to employees, and at follow-up we found that three employees had developed RADS after the release, and more than 100 employees reported symptoms of PTSD. Affected employees should be encouraged to report ongoing symptoms to their supervisor or to the plant health clinic for referral to appropriate care. Steps should be taken by the employer to ensure that health and safety messages are communicated effectively to everyone at risk, whatever their primary language or level of literacy.

RECOMMENDATIONS

On the basis of our findings, we recommend the actions listed below to create a more healthful workplace. We encourage the plant to use their labor-management health and safety committee to discuss the recommendations in this report and develop an action plan. Those involved in the work can best set priorities and assess the feasibility of our recommendations for the specific situation at the plant. Our recommendations are based on the hierarchy of controls approach (refer to Appendix C: Occupational Exposure Limits and Health Effects). This approach groups actions by their likely effectiveness in reducing or removing hazards. In most cases, the preferred approach is to eliminate hazardous materials or processes and install engineering controls to reduce exposure or shield employees. Until such controls are in place, or if they are not effective or feasible, administrative measures and/or personal protective equipment may be needed.

Elimination and Substitution

Elimination or substitution of a toxic/hazardous process material is a highly effective means for reducing hazards. Incorporating this strategy into the design or development phase of a project, commonly referred to as "prevention through design," is most effective because it reduces the need for additional controls in the future.

1. Consider using a less hazardous disinfectant. The United States Department of Agriculture, Food Safety and Inspection Service publishes and periodically updates Directive 7120.1, *Safe and Suitable Ingredients Used in the Production of Meat, Poultry, and Egg Products* [USDA 2012]. We recommend choosing the least hazardous, most effective disinfectants for each application from the lists in this directive.

Engineering Controls

Engineering controls reduce exposures to employees by removing the hazard from the process or placing a barrier between the hazard and the employee. Engineering controls are very effective at protecting employees without placing primary responsibility of implementation on the employee.

1. Investigate technology that may prevent future human error. We suggest finding unique fittings that will prevent connections from the filling station to the container.

2. Keep incompatible chemicals in different sized or different colored barrels to help keep from them being mixed up.

Administrative Controls

Administrative controls are management-dictated work practices and policies to reduce or prevent exposures to workplace hazards. The effectiveness of administrative changes in work practices for controlling workplace hazards is dependent on management commitment and employee acceptance. Regular monitoring and reinforcement are necessary to ensure that control policies and procedures are not circumvented in the name of convenience or production.

1. Ensure employee training programs regarding the hazardous chemicals used on-site and needed protective measures

Recommendations (continued)

comply with the upcoming changes in the OSHA hazard communication standard.

2. Establish evacuation plans for chemical releases which include rapidly conveying information on routes to take to evacuate and avoid the area where the chemical release occurred. This likely will include announcements over your public address system in appropriate languages. Practice these evacuation plans because employees need to know the proper evacuation routes from their workstation and feel that they are safe and effective.

3. Improve employee-management communication. This will be complicated because of the language barriers that are present in the plant. We recommend the following actions to address these important issues:

   - Provide details about the unintentional chlorine gas release (why it happened and what is being done to prevent future events) and the health risks of chlorine gas exposure. The Centers for Disease Control and Prevention has a fact sheet on chlorine that can be used (http://www.bt.cdc.gov/agent/chlorine/basics/facts.asp), as does the New Jersey Department of Health (http://web.doh.state.nj.us/rtkhsfs/factsheets.aspx?lan=spanish&alph=A&carcinogen=False&new=False#top).

   - Provide recommendations to employees about medical care post-exposure. We suggest seeking care from physicians trained in occupational and environmental medicine or toxicology. The employees we interviewed had received mixed messages about health risks from local physicians.

4. Continue the existing joint employee-management committee to address workplace safety and health issues. Bilingual employee representatives who can communicate in the employees' primary languages are important to the committee's success.

References

American Community Survey [2010]. Population of United States by People, Origin, Foreign and Native Born S0501 in 1 year. [http://www.census.gov/population/foreign/data/afftables_sub.html]. U.S. Census Bureau. Date accessed: September 2012.

REFERENCES
(CONTINUED)

American Psychiatric Association [2000]. Diagnostic and Statistical Manual of Mental Disorders. Rev. 4th ed. Washington, DC.

Arcury TA, Estrada JM, Quandt SA [2010]. Overcoming language and literacy barriers in safety and health training of agricultural workers. J Agromedicine 15(3):236–248.

Bisson JI [2007]. Post-traumatic stress disorder. BMJ 334(7597):789–793.

Brewin CR, Rose S, Andrews B, Green J, Tata P, McEvedy C, Turner S, Foa E [2002]. Brief screening instrument for post-traumatic stress disorder. Br J Psychiatry 181(Aug):158–162.

Brewin CR [2005]. Systematic review of screening instruments for adults at risk of PTSD. J Traum Stress 18(1):53–62.

Bureau of Labor Statistics [2011]. Current population survey. Employment and Earnings. Household data annual averages. 18. Employed persons by detailed industry, sex, race, and Hispanic or Latino ethnicity. Washington, DC: U.S. Department of Labor, Bureau of Labor Statistics. [http://www.bls.gov/cps/cpsa2010.pdf]. Date accessed: September 2012.

Das R, Blanc R [1993]. Chlorine gas exposure and the lung: a review. Toxic Industr Hlth 9(3):439–455.

Duncan MA, Drociuk D, Belflower-Thomas A, Van Sickle D, Gibson J, Younglood C, Daley WR [2011]. Follow-up assessment of health consequences after a chlorine release from a train derailment-Graniteville, SC, 2005. J Med Tox 7(1):85–91.

Grassi M, Rezzani C, Biino G, Marinoni A [2003]. Asthma-like symptoms assessment through ECRHS screening questionnaire scoring. J Clin Epidem 56(3):238–247.

Institute of Education Sciences, National Center for Educational Statistics, U.S. Department of Education [2003]. National assessment of adult literacy. [http://nces.ed.gov/naal/]. Date accessed: September 2012.

Johnson S, Ostendorf J [2010]. Hispanic employees in the workplace: higher rate of fatalities. AAOH 58(1):11–16.

References
(Continued)

Malo JL, L'archevêque J, Castellanos L, Lavoie K, Ghezzo H, Maghni K [2009]. Long-term outcomes of acute irritant-induced asthma. Am J Respir Crit Care Med 179(10):923–928.

OSHA [2012]. Safety and Health Topics. Hazard Communication, April 4, 2012. [http://www.osha.gov/dsg/hazcom/index.html]. Date accessed: September 2012.

Shakeri MS, Dick FD, Ayres JG [2008]. Which agents cause reactive airway dysfunction syndrome (RADS)? A systematic review. Occup Med 58(3):205–211.

USDA [2012]. Directive 7120.1: safe and suitable ingredients used in the production of meat, poultry, and egg products. [http://www.fsis.usda.gov/oppde/rdad/fsisdirectives/7120.1.pdf]. Date accessed: February 2013.

U.S. Government Accountability Office [2005]. Safety in the meat and poultry industry, while improving, could be further strengthened. Washington, DC: USGAO-05-96.

Wallerstein N [1992]. Health and safety education for workers with low-literacy or limited-English skills. Am J Ind Med 22(5):751–765.

Appendix A: Diagnostic Criteria for RADS and PTSD

The diagnostic criteria for RADS [Brooks et al. 1985] are listed below.
1. A documented absence of preceding respiratory complaints.

2. The onset of symptoms occurred after a single specific exposure incident or accident.

3. The exposure was to a gas, smoke, fume or vapor which was present in very high concentrations and had irritant qualities to its nature.

4. The onset of symptoms occurred within 24 hours after the exposure and persisted for at least 3 months.

5. Symptoms simulated asthma with cough, wheeze, and dyspnea predominating.

6. Pulmonary function tests may show airflow obstruction.

7. Methacholine challenge testing was positive.

8. Other types of pulmonary diseases were ruled out.

The diagnostic criteria for PTSD [American Psychiatric Association 2000] are listed below.
1. The person has been exposed to a traumatic event in which both of the following were present:
   a. The person has experienced, witnessed, or was confronted with an event or events that involved actual or threatened death or serious injury, or a threat to the physical integrity of oneself or others.
   b. The person's response involved intense fear, helplessness, or horror.
   Note: in children, this may be expressed instead by disorganized or agitated behavior

2. The traumatic event is persistently re-experienced in at least **one** of the following ways:
   a. Recurrent and intrusive distressing recollections of the event, including images, thoughts, or perceptions
   b. Recurrent distressing dreams of the event
   c. Acting or feeling as if the traumatic event were recurring (includes a sense of reliving the experience, illusions, hallucinations, and dissociative flashback episodes, including those that occur upon awakening or when intoxicated)
   d. Intense psychological distress at exposure to internal or external cues that symbolize or resemble an aspect of the traumatic event
   e. Physiologic reactivity on exposure to internal or external cues that symbolize or resemble an aspect of the traumatic event

3. Persistent avoidance of stimuli associated with the trauma and numbing of general responsiveness (not present before the trauma), as indicated by **three** (or more) of the following:
   a. Efforts to avoid thoughts, feelings, or conversations associated with the trauma
   b. Efforts to avoid activities, places, or people that arouse recollections of the trauma
   c. Inability to recall an important aspect of the trauma
   d. Markedly diminished interest or participation in significant activities
   e. Feeling of detachment or estrangement from others

f. Restricted range of affect (e.g., unable to have loving feelings)

g. Sense of a foreshortened future (e.g., does not expect to have a career, marriage, children, or a normal life span)

4. Persistent symptoms of increased arousal (not present before the trauma) as indicated by **two** (or more) of the following:

a. Difficulty falling or staying asleep

b. Irritability or outbursts of anger

c. Difficulty concentrating

d. Hypervigilance

e. Exaggerated startle response

5. Duration of the disturbance (symptoms in criteria 2, 3, and 4) is more than 1 month.

6. The disturbance causes clinically significant distress or impairment in social, occupational, or other important areas of functioning.

Specify if: Acute: if duration of symptoms is less than 3 months.

Chronic: if duration of symptoms is 3 months or more.

Specify if: With delayed onset: onset of symptoms at least 6 months after the stressor

References

American Psychiatric Association [2000]. Diagnostic and statistical manual of mental disorders. 4th rev. ed. Washington, DC.

Brooks SM, Weiss MA, Bernstein IL [1985]. Reactive airways dysfunction syndrome (RADS). Persistent asthma syndrome after high level irritant exposures. Chest 88(3):376–384.

APPENDIX B: METHACHOLINE CHALLENGE TESTING

Participants were evaluated by questionnaire, medical history, pulse, and blood pressure to determine suitability for spirometry. Participants who had a medical condition that restricted them from spirometry or methacholine challenge testing were not tested. We followed the algorithm shown below to test participants for bronchial hyperresponsiveness.

Methacholine Challenge Test Algorithm

1. **Do baseline spirometry**

2. a. **If baseline FEV1 ≥70% predicted** → Do methacholine challenge; after each concentration of methacholine, readminister spirometry

   if FEV1 is >80% of baseline FEV1 → go to next higher concentration of methacholine solution or stop if at last concentration.

   OR

   if FEV1 is below 80% of baseline FEV1 → administer bronchodilator and readminister spirometry after 10 minutes, if FEV1 is within 90% of baseline FEV1 subject is finished, otherwise administer bronchodilator again, wait 10 minutes and check spirometry again.

   OR

   b. **If baseline FEV1 <70% predicted** → administer bronchodilator and readminister spirometry after 10 minutes. We define reversible obstruction as an increase in FEV1 of 12% and at least 200 mL.

If, after all rounds of methacholine challenge, participants were unable to achieve an FEV1 below 80% of baseline, they were classified as nonresponders to the methacholine challenge test and classified as not having asthma. A positive methacholine challenge test (decrement of FEV1 below 80% of baseline) indicates bronchial hyperresponsiveness, consistent with asthma. Depending on the dose of methacholine, the test can indicate mild, moderate, and severe hyperresponsiveness. If during baseline spirometry they had a baseline less than 70% predicted FEV1, and responded to bronchodilators by improving 12% and at least 200 mL, then those participants were also classified as having bronchial hyperresponsiveness consistent with asthma. Otherwise, they were classified as not having asthma. Participants were notified in writing, in their primary language, of their test results.

Appendix C: Occupational Exposure Limits and Health Effects

In evaluating the hazards posed by workplace exposures, NIOSH investigators use both mandatory (legally enforceable) and recommended OELs for chemical, physical, and biological agents as a guide for making recommendations. OELs have been developed by federal agencies and safety and health organizations to prevent the occurrence of adverse health effects from workplace exposures. Generally, OELs suggest levels of exposure that most employees may be exposed to for up to 10 hours per day, 40 hours per week, for a working lifetime, without experiencing adverse health effects. However, not all employees will be protected from adverse health effects even if their exposures are maintained below these levels. A small percentage may experience adverse health effects because of individual susceptibility, a preexisting medical condition, and/or a hypersensitivity (allergy). In addition, some hazardous substances may act in combination with other workplace exposures, the general environment, or with medications or personal habits of the employee to produce adverse health effects even if the occupational exposures are controlled at the level set by the exposure limit. Also, some substances can be absorbed by direct contact with the skin and mucous membranes in addition to being inhaled, which contributes to the individual's overall exposure.

Most OELs are expressed as a TWA exposure. A TWA refers to the average exposure during a normal 8- to 10-hour workday. Some chemical substances and physical agents have recommended STEL or ceiling values where adverse health effects are caused by exposures over a short period. Unless otherwise noted, the STEL is a 15-minute TWA exposure that should not be exceeded at any time during a workday, and the ceiling limit is an exposure that should not be exceeded at any time.

In the United States, OELs have been established by federal agencies, professional organizations, state and local governments, and other entities. Some OELs are legally enforceable limits, while others are recommendations. The U.S. Department of Labor OSHA PELs (29 CFR 1910 [general industry]; 29 CFR 1926 [construction industry]; and 29 CFR 1917 [maritime industry]) are legal limits enforceable in workplaces covered under the Occupational Safety and Health Act of 1970. NIOSH RELs are recommendations based on a critical review of the scientific and technical information available on a given hazard and the adequacy of methods to identify and control the hazard. NIOSH RELs can be found in the NIOSH Pocket Guide to Chemical Hazards [NIOSH 2010]. NIOSH also recommends different types of risk management practices (e.g., engineering controls, safe work practices, employee education/ training, personal protective equipment, and exposure and medical monitoring) to minimize the risk of exposure and adverse health effects from these hazards. Other OELs that are commonly used and cited in the United States include the TLVs recommended by ACGIH, a professional organization, and the WEELs recommended by the American Industrial Hygiene Association, another professional organization. The TLVs and WEELs are developed by committee members of these associations from a review of the published, peer-reviewed literature. They are not consensus standards. ACGIH TLVs are considered voluntary exposure guidelines for use by industrial hygienists and others trained in this discipline "to assist in the control of health hazards" [ACGIH 2012]. WEELs have been established for some chemicals "when no other legal or authoritative limits exist" [AIHA 2012].

Outside the United States, OELs have been established by various agencies and organizations and include both legal and recommended limits. The Institut für Arbeitsschutz der Deutschen Gesetzlichen Unfallversicherung (IFA, Institute for Occupational Safety and Health of the German Social Accident

Insurance) maintains a database of international OELs from European Union member states, Canada (Québec), Japan, Switzerland, and the United States. The database, available at http://www.dguv.de/ifa/en/gestis/limit_values/index.jsp, contains international limits for over 1,500 hazardous substances and is updated periodically.

Employers should understand that not all hazardous chemicals have specific OSHA PELs, and for some agents the legally enforceable and recommended limits may not reflect current health-based information. However, an employer is still required by OSHA to protect its employees from hazards even in the absence of a specific OSHA PEL. OSHA requires an employer to furnish employees a place of employment free from recognized hazards that cause or are likely to cause death or serious physical harm [Occupational Safety and Health Act of 1970 (Public Law 91–596, sec. 5(a)(1))]. Thus, NIOSH investigators encourage employers to make use of other OELs when making risk assessments and risk management decisions to best protect the health of their employees. NIOSH investigators also encourage the use of the traditional hierarchy of controls approach to eliminate or minimize identified workplace hazards. This includes, in order of preference, the use of (1) substitution or elimination of the hazardous agent, (2) engineering controls (e.g., local exhaust ventilation, process enclosure, dilution ventilation), (3) administrative controls (e.g., limiting time of exposure, employee training, work practice changes, medical surveillance), and (4) personal protective equipment (e.g., respiratory protection, gloves, eye protection, hearing protection). Control banding, a qualitative risk assessment and risk management tool, is a complementary approach to protecting employee health that focuses resources on exposure controls by describing how a risk needs to be managed. Information on control banding is available at http://www.cdc.gov/niosh/topics/ctrlbanding/. This approach can be applied in situations where OELs have not been established or can be used to supplement the OELs, when available.

Below we provide the OELs for chlorine, as well as a discussion of the potential health effects from exposure to chlorine gas.

Chlorine

Chlorine is a greenish-yellow gas and has a pungent smell, with an odor threshold of approximately 0.3–0.5 ppm. Chlorine gas was the first chemical used in modern warfare. It was used by the Germans in Ypres, Belgium, on April 22, 1915, resulting in 5,000 pulmonary casualties [Evans 2004].

Chlorine is moderately water soluble, so it can enter the upper and lower respiratory tract and often affects mucus membranes, eyes, and the lower respiratory tract. It forms hydrochloric and hypochlorous acid upon contact with water in the eyes, mucus membranes, and lower respiratory tract [Das and Blanc 1993].

Table C1. Chlorine gas concentration and health effects

Concentration	Effect on human health
1–3 ppm	Mild irritation of mucous membranes
>5 ppm	Eye irritation
>15 ppm	Throat irritation
15–30 ppm	Cough, choking, burning
>50 ppm	Chemical pneumonitis
430 ppm	Death after 30 minutes exposure
>1000 ppm	Death within minutes

The current OSHA PEL for chlorine is 1 ppm (3 mg/m³) as a ceiling limit. A worker's exposure to chlorine shall at no time exceed this ceiling level [29 CFR 1910.1000, Table Z-1]. NIOSH has established a REL for chlorine of 0.5 ppm (1 5 mg/m³) as a TWA for up to a 10-hour workday and a 40-hour workweek and a STEL of 1 ppm (3 mg/m³) [NIOSH 1992]. The ACGIH TLV is 0.5 ppm (1.5 mg/m³) as a TWA for a normal 8-hour workday and a 40-hour workweek and a STEL of 1.0 ppm (2.9 mg/m³) for periods not to exceed 15 minutes. Exposures at the STEL concentration should not be repeated more than four times a day and should be separated by intervals of at least 60 minutes [ACGIH 2012].

References

ACGIH [2012]. 2012 TLVs® and BEIs®: threshold limit values for chemical substances and physical agents and biological exposure indices. Cincinnati, OH: American Conference of Governmental Industrial Hygienists.

AIHA [2012]. AIHA 2012 Emergency response planning guidelines (ERPG) & workplace environmental exposure levels (WEEL) handbook. Fairfax, VA: American Industrial Hygiene Association.

CFR. Code of Federal Regulations. Washington, DC: U.S. Government Printing Office, Office of the Federal Register.

Das R, Blanc R [1993]. Chlorine gas exposure and the lung: a review. Toxic Industr Hlth 9(3):439–455.

Evans RB [2004]. Chlorine: State of the Art. Lung 183(3):151–167.

NIOSH [1992]. Recommendations for occupational safety and health: compendium of policy documents and statements by Dames BL. Cincinnati, OH: U.S. Department of Health and Human Services, Centers for Disease Control and Prevention, National Institute for Occupational Safety and Health, DHHS (NIOSH) Publication No. 92-100.

NIOSH [2010]. NIOSH pocket guide to chemical hazards. Cincinnati, OH: U.S. Department of Health and Human Services, Centers for Disease Control and Prevention, National Institute for Occupational Safety and Health, DHHS (NIOSH) Publication No. 2010-168c. [http://www.cdc.gov/niosh/npg/]. Date accessed: September 2012.

Acknowledgments and Availability of Report

The Hazard Evaluations and Technical Assistance Branch (HETAB) of the National Institute for Occupational Safety and Health (NIOSH) conducts field investigations of possible health hazards in the workplace. These investigations are conducted under the authority of Section 20(a)(6) of the Occupational Safety and Health Act of 1970, 29 U.S.C. 669(a)(6) which authorizes the Secretary of Health and Human Services, following a written request from any employer or authorized representative of employees, to determine whether any substance normally found in the place of employment has potentially toxic effects in such concentrations as used or found. HETAB also provides, upon request, technical and consultative assistance to federal, state, and local agencies; labor; industry; and other groups or individuals to control occupational health hazards and to prevent related trauma and disease.

Mention of any company or product does not constitute endorsement by NIOSH. In addition, citations to websites external to NIOSH do not constitute NIOSH endorsement of the sponsoring organizations or their programs or products. Furthermore, NIOSH is not responsible for the content of these websites. All Web addresses referenced in this document were accessible as of the publication date.

This report was prepared by Francisco Meza, Charles Mueller, and Bradley King of HETAB. Field assistance was provided by Walter Alarcon, Diana Ceballos, Elizabeth Garza, Melody Kawamoto, Rachel Weintraub, Sandy Hainline, Williamina Bing, Jim Wilson, Ashley Whitlow, and Kenny Boaz. Health communication assistance was provided by Stefanie Evans. Editorial assistance was provided by Ellen Galloway. Desktop publishing was performed by Mary Winfree and Greg Hartle.

Copies of this report have been sent to employee and management representatives at the poultry plant, the state health department, and the Occupational Safety and Health Administration Regional Office. This report is not copyrighted and may be freely reproduced. The report may be viewed and printed at http://www.cdc.gov/niosh/hhe/. Copies may be purchased from the National Technical Information Service at 5825 Port Royal Road, Springfield, Virginia 22161.

www.ingramcontent.com/pod-product-compliance
Lightning Source LLC
Chambersburg PA
CBHW080933290526
45795CB00007BA/2735